GOD'S MEDICINE
HEALING
CONFESSIONS

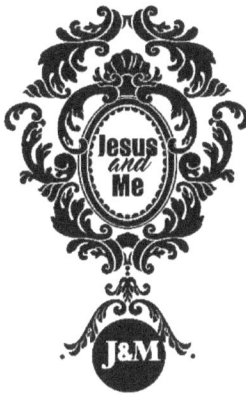

COMPILED BY

ELLEN A. CARTER

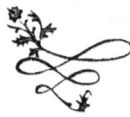

PRAYER:

Heavenly Father, I ask that your angels surround myself and my family members and protect us according to your word in Isaiah 54:17 as I declare NO weapons shall be formed against me and all my family shall prosper in the mighty name of Jesus!

I bind all Satan's evil spirits and demonic forces. I bind all king and princes of terrors. Remove all demonic entities and evil forces of nature, and drive them away from our spirits, mind, bodies, and souls.

I revoke any orders given to any of these demonic spirits and demonic forces concerning me and my family. I bind all demonic entities under the highest authority, our Lord Jesus!

Evil spirits, I loose you to go down to the pits of hell where you belong—to where Jesus Christ sends you. Your assignments, and influences in our lives are no more— completely broken in Jesus name!

By the blood of Jesus Christ, I declare broken and destroyed all spells, satanic rituals, Masonic and satanic blood covenants and sacrifices, evil wishes, and any type of curse-like judgments that have been sent our way and have been passed down through my family's generational bloodline. I loose them to Jesus Christ.

I ask forgiveness and renounce, all negative inner vows made by myself. I ask you Lord, Jesus Christ that you release me and mine from these vows and from any form of bondage that they may have held us in, in the mighty name of Jesus. Do not remember the iniquities of our forefathers or hold them against us. Instead, let Your compassion come quickly to meet us.

I now take the Sword of Spirit, which is the Word of God, and cut myself and my family members free. Free us from all generational curses, inherited sins, all personality traits, learned negative inner vows, all forms of spiritual, demonic and psychological ties. I cut all ties that are not of the Lord and put the blood of Jesus between us- back to the beginning of time and toward all present and future generations. By the Word of God, the Sword of the Spirit, and in the mighty name of Jesus Christ, I say that from now on, we are free, and we are now free indeed! We are now free to become the children of God as the Lord intended us to be. In my mighty name of Jesus. Amen!

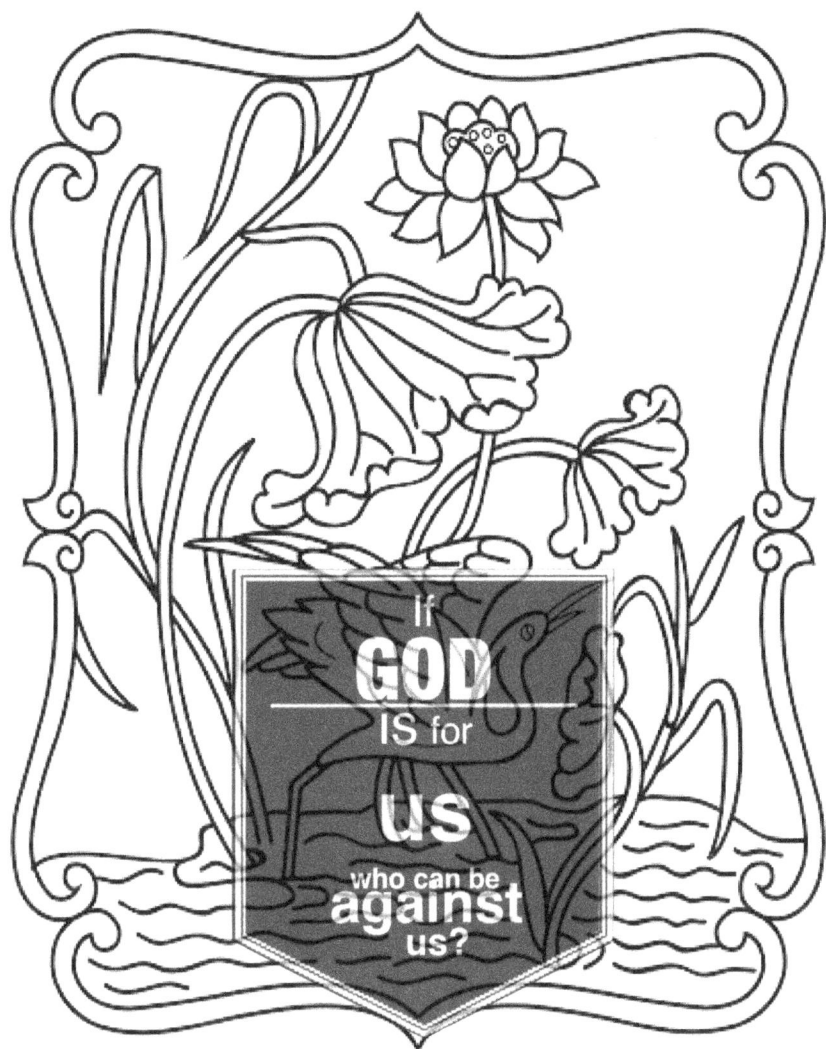

If
GOD
IS for

US

who can be
against
us?

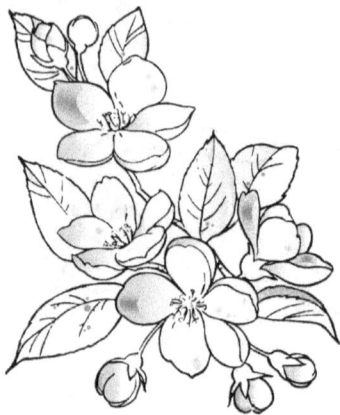

"Blessed is she who has believed that the Lord would fulfill what He has spoken to her!"

Luke 1:45

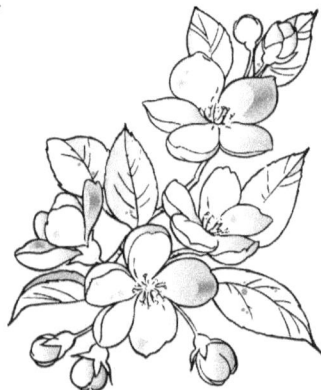

Dedication

This book is especially dedicated to the brave cancer fighters and survivors.

To my family—Josh, Mom, Mama, Kuya Alan, Roy and Jamie~It is those special moments of emotional connection with each one of you as my family where you give yourself in my time of need selflessly that I feel most loved—and for the most part, I can honestly say that the change was necessary for the better. But one of the most positive things it has brought is this new closeness and a greater appreciation for life and how important each one of you with deepest gratitude in so many levels. Even in this time of darkness and maybe times of uncertainty, its the love of Christ and the love from each one of you that drives out fear. I'm never alone knowing I got God with me nearer than ever before who will never leave me nor forsake me is the most loving and comforting feeling I have ever felt in the face of adversity. I love you all equally and I feel so blessed to have all of you in my life. God is good! To God be the glory!

Joyce Lomasang~ Just to let you know that God is still in control, Joyce. Let's continue to fight the good fight of faith! Troubles point out our weaknesses and prompt us to fully rely on God. We both know God can always bring good out of every situation whether in this life or the after life. What our spiritual enemy meant for bad, God always meant it for good to those who love Him— The God of all grace, who called us to His eternal glory in Christ Jesus. Love you, Joyce Lomasang! And of course ate Helen De Maya, stay beautiful and stay blessed always!

Silvia Diab- You are one strong fighter woman I know. You inspire me with your positive outlook in life.Thank you so much for taking the time to show you care. You have always been a positive individual who tries to be fair even at work. The only good thing about times of adversity is that you realized who your friends are. I just want to say "Thank you"

Allan and Sarah Balbon~ Thank you both so much for the love. For letting God's love shine through your hearts. Wonderful people like you make me realize just how much God loves me. I pray that God will bless both of you in so many ways more than your generous hearts can contain. May the LORD cause His face to shine upon the both of you always.

Dad and Oma- I love you both so much. I am so grateful that God has blessed me with a very special people in my life who makes me feel that I'm truly part of the family. I love you both so much more than you'll ever know.
To Mom and Danny- So grateful for the love and to be part of the family. Your thoughtful and caring ways truly warms my heart. Love you both.

To all others,I apologize if I miss to mention your names here... Love you all!!
Michelle & Julio Lara, Maureen & Jun Aves, Shiela & Carl Madriaga, Cheryl & Cliff Gaspar, Norman & Medik Chaves, Marvin & Ting-ting Chaves,Jeffrey & Yvonne Chaves, Kenneth & Marivic Chaves, Claudine & Ed Canosa, Christian & Beth, Ron & Jaylani Chaves, Arman & Liza Chaves, Glen & Faith Chaves, Anton Aldana. Jay & Claire Yap, Maybelle & Ramil Encarnado, **Ronnie & Carmen Chaves,Lino & Elvie Chaves, Carling & Norma Chaves, Nellie & Paquito Yap, Marissa & Mayo Gustillo,** Johanna & Jaybee Cruz, Joel and Karla Bautista, Mie & Chris Devers, Yosuke & Angela Carter, Jaime & John Sellers, Judy Carter, Johnny & Hyun-joo Carter, Adam & Alex McLaughlin. Eleonor Beltran, Aida Liwanag, Cynthia Lozania, Daniel Woube,Paul Bonaman,Tishara Day, Ana Curi, Genet Solomon, Joyce Carter, Clyde Ebo. Halina Hart, Mimi Soriano, Marjou Chabon Borlongan, Pastor Fred & Zinnia De la Rosa, Marino Olivieri,Pastor Herbert & Ingrid Ares.

Know Peace Know Jesus Know Peace Know Jesus Know Peace Know Jesus Know Peace Know Jesus Know Peace Know Jesus Know Peace Know Jesus Know Peace Know Jesus Know Peace Know Jesus

1 JOHN 4:4

"Ye are of God, little children, and have overcome them: because greater is he that is in you, than he that is in the world."

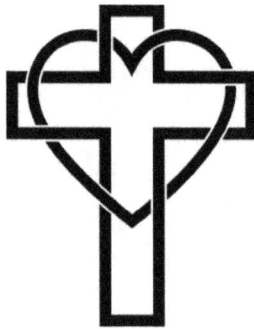

Psalm 30:2
"O LORD my God, I cried to You
for help, and You healed me."

INTRODUCTION

$\mathcal{H}$ello. Let me introduce myself to you:

I'm Ellen A. Carter. Please let me start my thoughts by telling you my personal story. I was diagnosed in October 2017, with breast cancer. I was given a six-month death sentence by my doctor. But instead of worrying, and throwing myself a pity party; instead of becoming fearful and depressed about my diagnosis, I put together these confessions of faith for myself and those who are faced with the same illness. I refuse any defeated thoughts as I channel my focus on Jesus. These confessions of faith remind me that our *strength* comes from **God**. I am also determined that I will not let the spirit of *fear* get the best of me, as I rely fully upon the power and guidance of the Holy Spirit in my life.

I decided that I will not let the troubles of this world, not even cancer, define me when I have a God who is alive; a God who is sitting on the Throne; who is in control. He is still the Giver of Life and the one who takes away. A God who created the Heaven and Earth, who can do the impossible, even beyond what doctors can't. I know Jesus is interceding for me in Heaven, and the Holy Spirit is guiding me on my journey. God is faithful and I am relying on His every Word. He is the one fighting our battles, rearranging things in our favor for eternal glory! This is the kind of conviction we all have in Jesus when we are fully surrendered to Him. The more I seek Him, the more I find Him because He draws nigh to those who draw nigh to Him, as I feel His strong presence in my life.

I have both joy and grief in the midst of trials which bring me closer to Him. Just like when I was grieving the loss of my dad, I learned that it takes years for the pain to ease. But in midst of the feeling of brokenness, I realized that God is the one who really provides consolation to those who mourn. Isn't it beautiful that God says He can give you beauty for ashes? I believe that the only way the wounded parts of our lives -- all kinds of them -- can be healed is when you give Him the agony of your brokenness. God can transform your hurt to healing once you hand Him all the broken pieces. It's the only way He can restore your life back to the way He designed it. He forgives and restores more than abundantly what has been taken. There is a beauty and blessing in our brokenness, in our pain, where God can appear and comfort us, that we may also find a profoundly renewed faith.

It is through the cracks of life that the Light of God enters into our hearts and into our souls. All these heart-wrenching experiences are the way that God transforms and takes away the unbelief left within us. It is His way to challenge us to become more resilient, powerful people of faith. He will refine us as silver is refined, test us as gold is tested. As He said, "They will call on My name, And I will answer them; I will say They are My people and they will say, The LORD is my God."

We have to know that God cannot allow unbelief to seep through our hearts which is a roadblock to our breakthroughs.

Every one of us build our life out of things and on a foundation. I built mine on a solid foundation of Jesus Christ. Every one of us will face storms of life one way or another. What we've build our life on, and out of will determine how well we weather the storm. It is only as we look unto Jesus with surrendered hearts that He will manifest His glory in our life.

As I am still walking in Life, I can only try to learn from what He is teaching me and ask Him to show me what more is needed from me. I am walking in deep waters, yet I am comforted by His grace knowing He is walking with me through it all.

I take this journey as a series of defining moments, and gratefully look to them as all the catalysts in my life that have moved me deeper and further in my spiritual journey. I try to always keep in mind that these are just simply necessary tools to mold me into having a more profound love -- a deep love for our Heavenly Father that may enable me to see His glory to glory as I walk in faith to faith. And while I'm in it, I strive to learn more about Him and welcome everything He is teaching me; and think about how much spiritual fruit this transformation will bring into my life!

I just knew I had to make a choice on how to react to things when death is staring me in the face, and what actions I will take: whether I will let myself be burned up and destroyed in the fire of afflictions, or rise from the ashes and soar.

"When the going gets tough, the tough get going". Just so I look up to Jesus in faith. Remember, the same power that raised up Jesus from the grave is living on the inside of you, as well as within me. Jesus said, "Let not your hearts be troubled. Believe in God; believe also in me."(John 14:1) Let us not fail to trust God fully for the problem we are facing. He is your strength as well as mine. There is a purpose for why I'm still alive today to write this to let you know He cares for you! And He does love YOU!

In weakness, there is always a glimmer of hope in JESUS, because He alone gives us hope—both for life now, and for eternity. And in our hope in Him, we find our strength and that includes the power not to have unholy turmoil of soul. Either way, as Christians, by death or life, we are victorious in Christ!

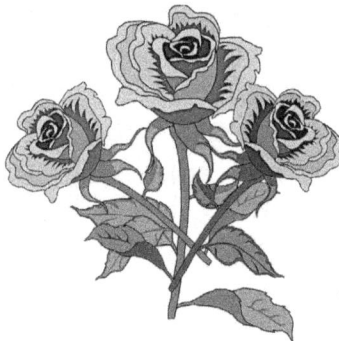

Jeremiah 1:12 (Amp.)
"Then the Lord said to me, "You have seen well, for I am [actively] watching over My word to fulfill it."

Thoughts to Ponder:

Do you believe what God said is true? Can you believe what God said He will do? Faith is a confident expectation. Unbelief in the promise of His Word forbids the benefit. Unbelief chokes the Word of God making it unfruitful. (Mark 4:19)
If you believe without a doubt, then you will find that you can operate in strong faith. Faith calls things in the spirit realm to the natural realm; and sometimes you have to speak it out loud and decree a thing that it shall be established unto you.

Fear can displace faith in our lives. Let us be like Abraham, who felt greater security in God's promises than he did in his circumstances. The same way, you have access to the gospel of Jesus Christ, where there is no record in the Bible turning away from anyone who came to Him for healing. God has a plan to bring healing to your life and all you have to do is stand on the promises of His Holy Word. Amen!

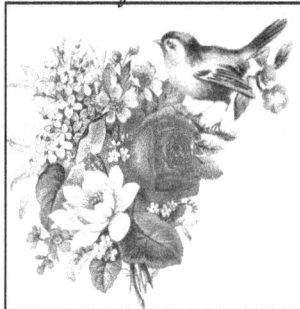

For Healing And Health Results
Speak Often And Speak A loudly!

*Just like when God said, "Let there be light",
there was light.* **Healing confession through
scriptures contain within them the capacity to
produce life and healing. Let's agree together**

*Proverbs 18:21 teaches us that there is the power
of life and death in our tongues. Essentially, this
means that the condition of our health is in the
words that we speak.*

*Let us learn how to speak words of faith that will
produce life and healing in our mortal bodies. It's
the knowledge of God's Word and believing them
that enables us to win the fight of faith against
sickness and disease. "Declare a thing, and it will
be done."(Job 22:28). Daily affirmation from
scripture encapsulate the message of our
guiding principles in action.*

Confession of faith can ultimately result not only in developing a more optimistic mindset, that is mapped out around God's Word, but as well as it rehearsed daily that affirms your love and trust for God as you internalized scripture that builds your faith.

Declaration of Faith
I receive the grace of God, which enables the power of God to work on my behalf.
I daily spend time reading God's healing Word, and my faith increases all the more.

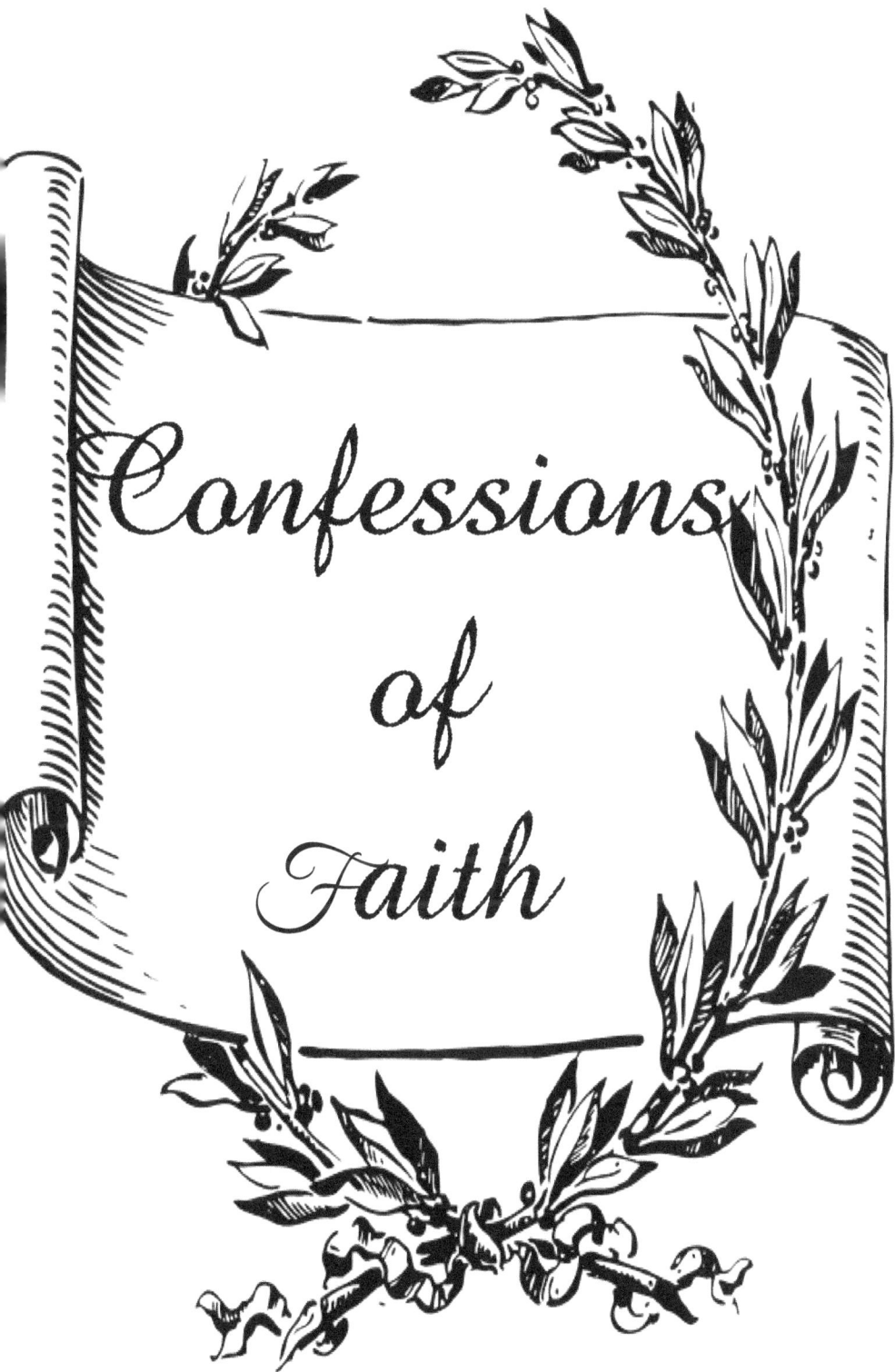

Confessions

of

Faith

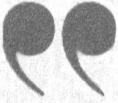

CONFESSION of FAITH:

Jesus is the Lord of my life. He is my personal Savior. He died on my behalf. He was my substitute. Jesus rose again from the dead. Satan has no power and dominion over me.

Philippians 2:11; Romans 10:9–10

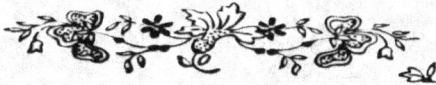

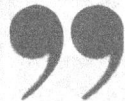

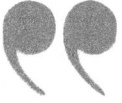

*F*or the **WORD** of **God** is quick and *powerful,* and *sharper* than any two-edged **SWORD**, piercing even to the dividing asunder of soul and spirit.

Hebrews 4:12

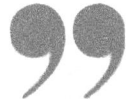

John 10:10

The thief cometh not, but for to steal, and to kill, and to destroy: I am come that they might have life, and that they might have it more abundantly.

CONFESSION of FAITH:

Jesus came that I may *have* life and have it in its **fullness.**

Exodus 15:26

And said, If thou wilt diligently hearken to the voice of the Lord thy God, and wilt do that which is right in his sight, and wilt give ear to his commandments, and keep all his statutes, I will put none of these diseases upon thee, which I have brought upon the Egyptians: for I am the Lord that healeth thee.

CONFESSION of FAITH:

I will *hearken* to the voice of the Lord my God and *give ear* to all His commandments and *keep* all His statutes for He is the Lord who heals me. Thank you, Lord, for healing me!

3 John 2

Beloved, I wish above all things that thou mayest prosper and be in health, even as thy soul prospereth.

CONFESSION of FAITH:

God desires that I *prosper* and be in health.

Acts 10:38

How God anointed Jesus of Nazareth with the Holy Ghost and with power: who went about doing good, and healing all that were oppressed of the devil; for God was with him.

CONFESSION of FAITH:

Jesus is the Healer of my soul; Satan is the oppressor. God anointed Jesus of Nazareth with the Holy Spirit and with power, Who went about doing good and healing all that were oppressed by the devil.

Proverbs 4:20–21

My son, attend to my words; incline thine ear unto My sayings. Let them not depart from thine eyes; keep them in the midst of thine heart for they are life unto those that find them, and health to all their flesh.

CONFESSION of FAITH:

Father, I will give attention to Your Words; I will incline my ear unto Your sayings. I will not let them depart from my sight and I will keep them within my heart. They are *life* to me for I have found them, and they are *health*, *healing* and medicine to all my flesh.

Deuteronomy 7:15

And the Lord will take away from thee all sickness, and will put none of the evil diseases of Egypt, which thou knowest, upon thee; but will lay them upon all them that hate thee.

CONFESSION of FAITH:

I am protected from all sickness and disease because all the sickness and disease of this world *were placed* on Jesus for me on Calvary's cross. Your Word, O Lord, will not return void but will accomplish what it was sent to do. Thank You, FATHER GOD, for taking away all sickness from me.

Hebrews 13:6

So that we may boldly say, The Lord is my helper, and I will not fear what man shall do unto me.

CONFESSION of FAITH:

The Lord is my helper, I will not be afraid nor be dismayed.
In God, I trust!

Christ hath redeemed us from the curse of the law, being made a curse for us: for it is written, Cursed is every one that hangeth on a tree:
That the blessing of Abraham might come on the Gentiles through Jesus Christ; that we might receive the promise of the Spirit through faith. Brethren, I speak after the manner of men; Though it be but a man's covenant, yet if it be confirmed, no man disannulleth, or addeth thereto.

CONFESSION of FAITH:

I am redeemed from all the curse of the Law since Jesus became a curse for me. I will not tolerate these curses for they are not in my new covenant in Christ, established in the righteousness of God. I refuse to allow the curses of the law to come on my body, for Christ already bought me with His blood and made me free from the law.

Joel 3:10

*B*eat your plowshares into swords and your pruninghooks into spears: let the weak say, I am strong.

*C*ONFESSION of FAITH:

*L*et the weak say, "I am strong." **I am strong** *in the* **Lord**. It's what the **Lord** has done in me.

Isaiah 33:24

And the inhabitant shall not say, I am sick: the people that dwell therein shall be forgiven their iniquity.

CONFESSION of FAITH:

The inhabitant will not say, I am sick. Therefore, I will NOT say it. I will only say what God has said in His Word in 1 Peter 2:24: By His wounds, I have been healed! For I have faith in His Word. **To God be the glory!!**

Mark 11:23

For verily I say unto you, That whosoever shall say unto this mountain, Be thou removed, and be thou cast into the sea; and shall not doubt in his heart, but shall believe that those things which he saith shall come to pass; he shall have whatsoever he saith.

CONFESSION of FAITH:

I do NOT doubt in my heart but believe that those things God says will come to pass, I also believe I will have whatever I say according to His Word. Therefore, the mountain of sickness, be removed from me, now! Be cast into the sea. Go now, spirit of infirmity! You have no place in me! You must as I command you in the name of Jesus!

Joshua 14:10–11

And now, behold, the Lord hath kept me alive, as he said, these forty and five years, even since the Lord spake this word unto Moses, while the children of Israel wandered in the wilderness: and now, lo, I am this day fourscore and five years old.

CONFESSION of FAITH:

The same Spirit who raised Jesus from the grave has given life to my body, spirit, and soul. That eternal life of God gives me strength and vigor for each new day whatever my age.

-PRAY THIS-

LORD JESUS, FORGIVE ME FOR ALL MY SINS THAT OPENED THE DOORS TO THE SPIRIT OF INFIRMITY. I REPENT OF THEM NOW! LORD, I FORGIVE THOSE WHO HAVE OFFENDED ME!I BIND AND CAST OUT ALL BITTERNESS AND RESENTMENT CONCERNING THEM! I BLESS THOSE THAT CURSE ME! THANK YOU JESUS FOR HEARING ME AND FORGIVING ME OF MY UNFORGIVENESS! IN JESUS' NAME I BIND YOU SATAN AND YOUR DEMONIC SPIRITS OF INFIRMITY AND DEATH! I CAST YOU OUT NOW IN JESUS' NAME! I BIND AND CAST OUT THE ILLNESSES OF_____

I PUT THE BLOOD OF JESUS AT THE ROOT AT WHICH THEY CAME IN. I CLOSE THOSE DOORS NOW! SEALED THEM WITH THE BLOOD OF JESUS! I SEND THEM TO JESUS FOR JUDGEMENT AND FORBID THEM TO COME BACK. SATAN YOU AND YOUR MINIONS; DEMONIC FORCES ARE ALREADY DEFEATED! GO NOW!!! LEAVE IN THE NAME OF JESUS! *I LOOSE NOW UPON MYSELF: HEALTH AND STRENGTH* INSTEAD OF SICKNESS AND DISEASE! I LOOSE THE HEALING POWER OF JESUS CHRIST OF NAZARETH! *I LOOSE THE HOLY SPIRIT TO HEAL CLEANSE, AND PURIFY AND FALL AFRESH ON ME! I LOOSE YOUR ANOINTING POWER ON ME, MY LORD JESUS.AMEN!*

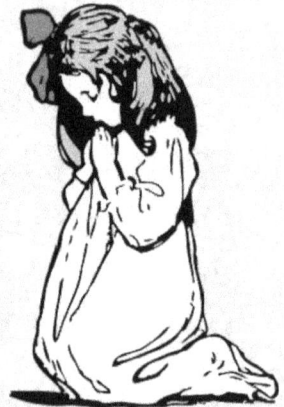

Luke 10:19

Behold, I give unto you power to tread on serpents and scorpions, and over all the power of the enemy: and nothing shall by any means hurt you.

CONFESSION of FAITH:

I have the power to tread on serpents and scorpions, and over all the power of the enemy: and nothing shall by any means hurt me through the blood of my Redeemer, Jesus Christ!

John 6:63

*I*t is the spirit that quickeneth; the flesh profiteth nothing: the words that I speak unto you, they are spirit, and they are life.

CONFESSION of FAITH:

*T*herefore, I will speak words of life. Jesus says His words are life in John 6:63 so I will speak them.

Job 5:26

Thou shalt come to thy grave in a full age, like as a shock of corn cometh in in his season.

CONFESSION of FAITH:

Father, I am going to live my life to the fullest, and if I go to the grave and should Jesus tarry, it will be at a very old age, full of vigor, vitality, and strength just like sheaves of grain harvested at harvest time.

Luke 8:11

Now the parable is this: The seed is the Word of God.

CONFESSION of FAITH:

When I speak God's Word I am planting good seed in my life.

Proverbs 18:21

Death and life are in the power of the tongue: and they that love it shall eat the fruit thereof.

CONFESSION of FAITH:

Since death and life are in the power of the tongue—therefore, I will only speak words of life, just as Jesus says in John 6:63.

Hebrews 10:23

Let us hold fast the profession of our faith without wavering; (for HE is faithful that promised;)

Hebrews 4:14

Seeing then that we have a great high priest, that is passed into the heavens, Jesus the Son of God, let us hold fast our profession.

CONFESSION of FAITH:

I will hold fast to the confession of God's Word without wavering, for He Who promised is faithful.

Romans 4:20,21

He staggered not at the promise of God through unbelief; but was strong in faith, giving glory to God;

CONFESSION of FAITH:

I do not waver at the promise of God through unbelief. God's promises never falter. He is not a man, that He should lie. I am fully convinced that what He has promised, He is also able to perform.

Romans 4:19 (Amp.)

He did not weaken in faith when he considered the [utter] impotence of his own body, which was as good as dead...

2 Corinthians 5:7

For we walk by faith, not by sight.

CONFESSION of FAITH:

I am not weak in faith, so I do not consider my own body above what God has said. I'm not moved by what I feel. I'm not moved by what I see. For I walk by faith not by sight. Yes, I'm moved only by what I believe. I believe the Word of God.

Proverbs 16:24

Pleasant words are as an honeycomb, sweet to the soul, and health to the bones.

CONFESSION of FAITH:

Pleasant words are health, healing and medicine to my bones. It is sweet to the soul.

Acts 20:32

And now, brethren, I commend you to God, and to the word of his grace, which is able to build you up, and to give you an inheritance among all them which are sanctified.

CONFESSION of FAITH:

God's Word of grace builds me up, and it gives me my inheritance among all them which are sanctified.

Galatians 5:13

For, brethren, ye have been called unto liberty; only use not liberty for an occasion to the flesh, but by love serve one another.

John 8:31–32

Then said Jesus to those Jews which believed in him, If ye continue in my word, then are ye my disciples indeed;And ye shall know the truth, and the truth shall make you free.

CONFESSION of FAITH:

I have been called to freedom. Jesus says that if I continue in His Word, then I will know the truth, and the truth shall set me free. I am free indeed! I am on God's team!

Therefore if any man be in Christ, he is a new creature: old things are passed away; behold, all things are become new.

CONFESSION of FAITH:

I am a new creation in Christ. Old things have passed away. All things have become new and all things are of God.

Romans 8:36–37

As it is written, For thy sake we are killed all the day long; we are accounted as sheep for the slaughter. Nay, in all these things we are more than conquerors through Him that loved us.

CONFESSION of FAITH:

Even though I am killed; all day long accounted as sheep for the slaughter, Nay, in all these things overwhelming *victory* is mine through **Christ** who loved me.

Philippians 1:6

Being confident of this very thing, that he which hath begun a good work in you will perform it until the day of Jesus Christ:

Confession of Faith:

I am confident of this, that He who began a good work in me will carry it on to completion until the day of Jesus Christ.

Ephesians 2:10

For we are his workmanship, created in Christ Jesus unto good works, which God hath before ordained that we should walk in them.

CONFESSION of FAITH:

I am God's workmanship, created in Christ Jesus. I am taking the path He ordained. I am saved by grace. I am walking in His will and Divine decree through the blood of my Savior, Jesus Christ.

But the Lord is faithful, who shall establish you, and keep you from evil.

CONFESSION of FAITH:

Lord you are faithful! Thank you for giving me strength and setting me on a firm foundation and guarding my soul from the evil one.

And ye are complete in **Him**, which is the head of all principality and power:

CONFESSION of FAITH:

I am complete in Jesus, Who is the head of all rulers, power and authority.

What? know ye not that your body is the temple of the Holy Ghost which is in you, which ye have of God, and ye are not your own?

For ye are **bought** with a price: therefore glorify God in your body, and in your spirit, which are God's.

CONFESSION of FAITH:

My body is a temple of the Holy Spirit. When I receive Christ, the Holy Spirit lives in me, and I am not my own. I am bought at a price. Therefore, I will glorify God in my body and my spirit which are God's.

I beseech you therefore, brethren, by the mercies of God, that ye present your bodies a living sacrifice, holy, and acceptable unto God, which is your reasonable service.

CONFESSION of FAITH:

I present my body to God as a living sacrifice, holy and acceptable.

Galatians 3:13

Christ hath redeemed us from the curse of the law, being made a curse for us: for it is written, Cursed is every one that hangeth on a tree:

Matthew 16:19

And I will give unto thee the keys of the kingdom of heaven: and whatsoever thou shalt bind on earth shall be bound in heaven: and whatsoever thou shalt loose on earth shall be loosed in heaven.

CONFESSION of FAITH:

Christ has redeemed me from the curse of the law, which includes all sickness. So, I forbid all form of sickness and disease in my body. Every germ or any virus that touches my body dies instantly by the blood of Jesus. Every cell, and organ, every member and system of my body functions perfectly, and I forbid any disruption and malfunction in the authority of Jesus Christ who already took the chastisement of my sins.

Psalm 27:1

The Lord is my light and my salvation; whom shall I fear? The Lord is the strength of my life; of whom shall I be afraid?

CONFESSION of FAITH:

The Lord is the strength of my life. Of whom shall I be afraid? I am in His good hands. Nothing can shake me, nor break me because I know You are in control. My hope is in You Lord, I put my trust in You!

Ephesians 6:10

Finally, my brethren, be strong in the Lord, and in the power of **His** might.

CONFESSION of FAITH:

I am strong in the Lord and in the power of His might. I have the victory in Christ!

Mark 9:23

Jesus said unto him, If thou canst believe, all things are possible to him that believeth.

CONFESSION of FAITH:

**I am a believer of Christ.
All things are possible to me!**

1 John 4:4

Ye are of God, little children, and have overcome them: because **greater** is **He** that is in **you,** than he that is in the world.

CONFESSION of FAITH:

Greater is He that is in me,
(The Holy Spirit who lives in me) than he (the defeated foe) who is in the world (the enemy who is the author of sickness.)

Giving **thanks unto the Father**, which hath made us meet to be partakers of the inheritance of the saints in light:Who hath delivered us from the power of darkness, and hath translated us into the kingdom of his dear Son:In whom we have redemption through his blood, even the forgiveness of sins:

CONFESSION of FAITH:

Thank you, Father, that Thou has made me able to be a partaker of my inheritance. Thank you that you delivered me from the authority of darkness, and have translated me into the kingdom of Your Son Jesus Christ, in Whom I have my redemption through His blood. Thank Lord, for the forgiveness of sins. Amen!

And they overcame him by the blood of the Lamb, and by the word of their testimony; and they loved not their lives unto the death.

CONFESSION of FAITH:

I am an overcomer, and I overcome through the blood of the Lamb and the word of my *testimony*.

James 4:7

Submit yourselves therefore to God. Resist the devil, and he will flee from you.

CONFESSION of FAITH:

I am not only a believer but an overcomer! I have submitted to God by being submissive to His Word. **God** is the one fighting my battle and the devil has no choice but to flee from me because I resist him with every fiber of my being in the supreme authority of my Savior and my High Priest, Jesus Christ!

Isaiah 54:17

No weapon that is formed against thee shall prosper; and **every tongue** that shall rise against thee in judgment thou shalt **condemn.** This is the heritage of the servants of the Lord, and their righteousness is of me, saith the Lord.

CONFESSION of FAITH:

No weapon that is formed against me shall prosper, and every tongue which rises against me in judgment, I will condemn. This is my heritage as a servant of the Lord, and my righteousness is from you, O Lord, of hosts.

Ephesians 4:32

And be ye kind one to another, tenderhearted, forgiving one another, even as God for Christ's sake hath forgiven you.

CONFESSION of FAITH:

I forgive others freely as God has forgiven me. I don't hold anything against anyone.

1 Peter 3:9

Not rendering evil for evil, or railing for railing: but contrariwise blessing; knowing that ye are thereunto called, that ye should inherit a blessing.

CONFESSION of FAITH:

I do not return evil for evil, but on the contrary, bless, for this I have been called that I may obtain a blessing. Amen!

Psalm 91:1

He that dwelleth in the secret place of the most High shall abide under the shadow of the Almighty.

CONFESSION of FAITH:

I dwell in the secret place of the most High and abide under the shadow of the **Almighty God**.

*F*or he that will love life, and see good days, let him refrain his tongue from evil, and his lips that they speak no guile:

*C*ONFESSION of FAITH:

I **refrain** my tongue from evil. I turn away from evil and do good. I **seek** peace and pursue it. So I will love the life God has given me and see good days.

Casting all your care upon him; for **He** careth for you.

CONFESSION of FAITH:

I have cast all my cares on the Lord, for He cares for me. I refuse any doubt, fear or worry about anything.

And ye shall serve the Lord your God, and he shall bless thy bread, and thy water; and I will take sickness away from the midst of thee.

CONFESSION of FAITH:

I serve the Lord my God, and He blesses my bread, and my water, and He has taken sickness away from me. Jesus took all my infirmities and bore all my sicknesses away. Thank you, Lord, for healing me!

Psalm 86:15

But thou, O Lord, art a God full of compassion, and gracious, long suffering, and plenteous in mercy and truth.

CONFESSION of FAITH:

Thank you, O Lord, that you are a God full of compassion, and gracious, long suffering and abundant in mercy and truth.

Isaiah 53:4

Surely **HE** hath borne our griefs, and carried our sorrows: yet we did esteem him stricken, smitten of God, and afflicted.

1 Peter 2:24

Who his own self bare our sins in his own body on the tree, that we, being dead to sins, should live unto righteousness: by whose stripes ye were healed.

CONFESSION of FAITH:

Thank you, O Lord, that you have borne my sicknesses and carried my pains. Jesus was wounded for my transgressions. He was bruised for my iniquities. The chastisement for my sin and peace was upon Him, and by His wounds, I am healed!

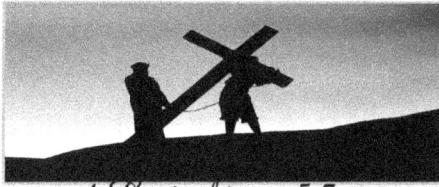

1 Corinthians 5:7

$\mathcal{P}$urge out therefore the old leaven, that ye may be a new lump, as ye are unleavened. For even Christ our passover is sacrificed for us:

$\mathcal{C}$ONFESSION of FAITH:

Jesus Christ my Passover was sacrificed for me. So all sickness and death has to pass over me and my household.

Deuteronomy 7:15

And the Lord will take away from thee all sickness, and will put none of the evil diseases of Egypt, which thou knowest, upon thee; but will lay them upon all them that hate thee.

CONFESSION of FAITH:

I thank you, Lord, that you have taken away from me all sickness and have clothed me with your grace and mercy. Thank you, Lord, for healing me.

O LORD my God, I cried unto thee, and thou hast healed me.

CONFESSION of FAITH:

Lord my God, I thank you that when I cried out to You, You restored my health.

Psalm 107:20

He sent his word, and healed them, and delivered them from their destructions.

.

CONFESSION of FAITH:

God sent His Word and healed me, and delivered me from destruction. Thank you, Lord, for healing me!

There shall be nothing that cast their young, nor be barren; in thy land: the number of thy days I will fulfill.

CONFESSION of FAITH:

The number of my days God will fulfill.

Psalm 103:1–5

Bless the Lord, O my soul: and all that is within me, bless his holy name. Bless the Lord, O my soul, and forget not all his benefits: Who forgiveth all thine iniquities; who healeth all thy diseases; Who redeemeth thy life from destruction; Who crowneth thee with lovingkindness and tender mercies; Who satisfieth thy mouth with good things; so that thy youth is renewed like the eagle's.

CONFESSION of FAITH:

Bless the Lord, O my soul: and all that is within me, bless His Holy Name! Bless the Lord, O my soul, and let me forget not all His benefits: Who *forgives* all my iniquities; Who heals all my diseases; Who redeems my life from destruction; the One Who crowns me with lovingkindness and tender mercies; Who satisfies my mouth with good things, so that my youth is renewed like the eagle's.

Matthew 28:18–19

And Jesus came and spake unto them, saying, All power is given unto me in heaven and in earth.

Luke 10:19

Behold, I give unto you power to tread on serpents and scorpions, and over all the power of the enemy: and nothing shall by any means hurt you.

Jesus came and spoke saying, "All authority (power) has been given unto me in heaven and on earth, and nothing shall by any means hurt me because I have the Spirit of God who lives in me."

According as his divine power hath given unto us all things that pertain unto life and godliness, through the knowledge of him that hath called us to glory and virtue.

CONFESSION of FAITH:

God's divine power has bestowed upon me all things that pertain unto life and godliness, through the knowledge of Him through which He has given to me exceedingly great and precious promises.

1 John 3:8

He that committeth sin is of the devil; for the devil sinneth from the beginning. For this purpose the Son of God was manifested, that he might destroy the works of the devil.

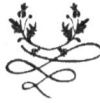

CONFESSION of FAITH:

For this purpose the Son of God was manifested: that He might destroy the works of the devil. And by this, I am commanding sickness to leave in my body now in Jesus' name!

That ye be not slothful, but followers of them who through faith and patience inherit the promises.

CONFESSION of FAITH:

Because of my faith and patience that pleases you, O Lord, I now inherit Your promises! Indeed, You are the source of my faith.

Job 22:28

Thou shalt also decree a thing, and it shall be established unto thee: and the light shall shine upon thy ways.

CONFESSION of FAITH:

Lord, Your word says I can declare truth and it will come to pass for me. Therefore, if I speak that I am healed, my future is bright. I believe in Your Word— and you light my path. Thank you, Lord!

The angel of the Lord encampeth round about them that fear him, and delivereth them. O taste and see that the Lord is good: blessed is the man that trusteth in him. O fear the Lord, ye his saints: for there is no want to them that fear him.The young lions do lack, and suffer hunger: but they that seek the Lord shall not want any good thing.

CONFESSION of FAITH:

Father thank you that when I cry out for help you hear me, you rescue me from all my troubles and I refuse to have my spirit crushed. Father, I respect your ways, therefore the angels encamp about me and deliver me, and I will never lack any good thing.

*M*any are the afflictions of the righteous: but the Lord delivereth him out of them all. He keepeth all his bones: not one of them is broken.

*C*ONFESSION of FAITH:

*F*ather, thank you that I am the righteousness of God, and I am delivered from every trouble or oppression from the enemy because you rescue me. You protect me from harm, and not one of my bones is broken. Thank you, Lord, that you deliver me from all my pain and afflictions.

Psalm 42:11

Why art thou cast down, O my soul? and why art thou disquieted within me? hope thou in God: for I shall yet praise him, who is the health of my countenance, and my God.

CONFESSION of FAITH:

Father God, I'am not discouraged or sad, because I put my hope in You. I praise and worship You, O Lord, my God.

Psalm 91:14–16

Because he hath set his love upon me, therefore will I deliver him: I will set him on high, because he hath known my name. He shall call upon me, and I will answer him: I will be with him in trouble; I will deliver him, and honour him. With long life will I satisfy him, and shew him my salvation

CONFESSION of FAITH:

Father, because I know you, I set my love upon you. You deliver me, and set me on high because I know your name— when I call upon You, You answer me. You are with me in trouble; You deliver me and honor me — You satisfy me, Lord, with long life and show me your salvation in every area of my life. Thank you, Jesus, for your faithfulness.

Bless the Lord, O my soul: and all that is within me, bless His holy name. Bless the Lord, O my soul, and forget not all His benefits: Who forgiveth all thine iniquities; Who healeth all thy diseases; Who redeemeth thy life from destruction; Who crowneth thee with lovingkindness and tender mercies;
Who satisfieth thy mouth with good things; so that thy youth is renewed like the eagle's. The Lord executeth righteousness and judgment for all that are oppressed.

CONFESSION of FAITH:

I bless the Lord with my soul and I do not forget any of His benefits, for He has forgiven all my sins and iniquities, and He has healed all my diseases. Thank you, Lord for healing me!

*H*e sent his word, and healed them, and delivered them from their destructions.

*C*ONFESSION of FAITH:

*F*ather, I thank you that you sent your Word and healed me, and delivered me from all destruction— even at the pit of death.

For thou hast girded me with strength unto the battle: thou hast subdued under me those that rose up against me.

CONFESSION of FAITH:

Thank you Lord, for arming me with strength and making my way perfect, and subduing under me those that rose up against me.

Psalm 27:5

For in the time of trouble He shall hide me in his pavilion: in the secret of his tabernacle shall he hide me; he shall set me up upon a rock.

CONFESSION of FAITH:

Thank you Lord, for hiding me in Your sanctuary!

Psalm 91:4

He shall cover thee with His feathers, and under His wings shalt thou trust: His truth shall be thy shield and buckler.

CONFESSION of FAITH:

Thank you my God, that You cover me with Your feathers. Under Your wings I find refuge. Your faithfulness and truth is my shield and buckler.

Thou art the God that doest wonders: thou hast declared thy strength among the people.

CONFESSION of FAITH:

Thank you, Lord, that You are the God of wonders. You are indeed a performing miracle God in me. You display Your power and You are the source of my strength.

Psalm 116:8

For thou hast delivered my soul from death, mine eyes from tears, and my feet from falling.

CONFESSION of FAITH:

Thank you, Lord, for delivering me from death, my eyes from tears, and my feet from stumbling.

Psalm 118:17

I shall not die, but live, and declare the works of the Lord..

CONFESSION of FAITH:

I shall not die, but live and declare the works of the Lord.

So shall my word be that goeth forth out of my mouth: it shall not return unto me void, but it shall accomplish that which I please, and it shall prosper in the thing whereto I sent it.

Confession of Faith:

I believe the Word of God with all my heart. My healing words of faith will not return to me empty in Jesus' name!

Psalm 138:3

He giveth power to the faint; and to them that have no might he increaseth strength.

Confession of Faith:

I thank you, Lord, for giving me strength when I'm weary, and increasing power when I have no might. You are the source of everything, and there is no other like you, Lord!

In the day when I cried thou answeredst me, and strengthenedst me with strength in my soul.

CONFESSION of FAITH:

Lord, I thank you that you answer me when I cry out to you, and You have made me bold with strength in my soul.
You are my faithful God!

For verily I say unto you, That whosoever shall say unto this mountain, Be thou removed, and be thou cast into the sea; and shall not doubt in his heart, but shall believe that those things which He saith shall come to pass; he shall have whatsoever he saith.

CONFESSION of FAITH:

I do NOT doubt in my heart but believe that those things God says will come to pass, I also believe I will have whatever I say through the blood of Jesus. Therefore, the mountain of sickness, be removed from me, now! Be cast into the sea. Go now, spirit of infirmity! You have no place in me! You must as I command you in the name of Jesus!

Who His own self bare our sins in His own body on the tree, that we, being dead to sins, should live unto righteousness: by whose stripes ye were healed.

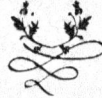

CONFESSION of FAITH:

Thank you, Lord, for fulfilling what You have spoken. By Jesus' stripes, I have now received my complete healing.

Mark 11:24

Therefore I say unto you, what things soever ye desire, when you pray, believe that you receive them, and you shall have them.

Psalm 107:20

He sent his word, and healed them, and delivered them from their destructions.

CONFESSION of FAITH:

Thank you, Lord, for You have healed me. I received it because I believed it! You sent Your Word and I am healed! By the Word which proceedeth out of Your mouth, I am restored from destruction!

Matthew 8:13

And Jesus said unto the centurion, Go thy way; and as thou hast believed, so be it done unto thee. And his servant was healed in the selfsame hour.

CONFESSION of FAITH:

Thank you, Jesus, that you destroyed the works of the devil, which were diseases, sicknesses, and bodily infirmities; therefore, all the works of the devil upon my body are destroyed and I have perfect health in Jesus name!

Isaiah 41:10

Looking unto Jesus the author and finisher of our faith; who for the joy that was set before him endured the cross, despising the shame, and is set down at the right hand of the throne of God.

Luke 10:19, Genesis 1:28

Behold, I give unto you power to tread on serpents and scorpions, and over all the power of the enemy: and nothing shall by any means hurt you.

CONFESSION of FAITH:

Jesus is in me, and He is the Author and Finisher of my faith. As a child of God, I have been given the authority and dominion over every living thing and overall disease and sickness— all power of the enemy. Nothing shall by any means hurt me. I command the spirit of infirmity to obey and leave in Jesus name!

John 1:12

*B*ut as many as received Him, to them gave He power to become the sons of God, even to them that believe on His name:

CONFESSION of FAITH:

I am His Son/Daughter of the most highest!

Isaiah 43:18–19

And if children, then heirs; heirs of God, and joint-heirs with Christ; if so be that we suffer with him, that we may be also glorified together.

CONFESSION of FAITH:

I am an heir of God and joint heirs with Christ. If so be that I suffer with Him, that I may be also glorified together.

*R*emember ye not the former things, neither consider the things of old. Behold, I will do a new thing; now it shall spring forth; shall ye not know it? I will even make a way in the wilderness, and rivers in the desert..V. 21This people have I formed for myself; they shall shew forth my praise.

*C*ONFESSION of FAITH:

I am being called by the God of Heaven and Earth, Who will do a new thing; Who calls me to not forget that all is nothing compared to what He is going to do. "For I am going to do something new." See, I have already begun!
And I say, "I see it, Lord! You are making a pathway through the wilderness. I now see clearly and recognize and discern the connections that You orchestrated in my life that are summoning me from one level to another, from glory to glory that I may grow from faith to faith— from one season to the next, that I may show forth Your praise!

Make This Strong Declaration.

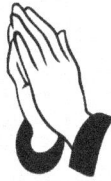

In the name of Jesus, I release myself from the enemy's attacks upon my physical well-being.
In the name of Jesus, I receive the healing and health that is God's provision for me and for my family. I stand now in the freedom from sickness that Jesus purchased for me on the calvary's cross. Healing and transformation I now experience through faith, in the name of, Jesus! Thank you, Lord, I am now healed. Amen.

"***Rejoice*** always, pray without ceasing,"

1 Thessalonians 5:16-17

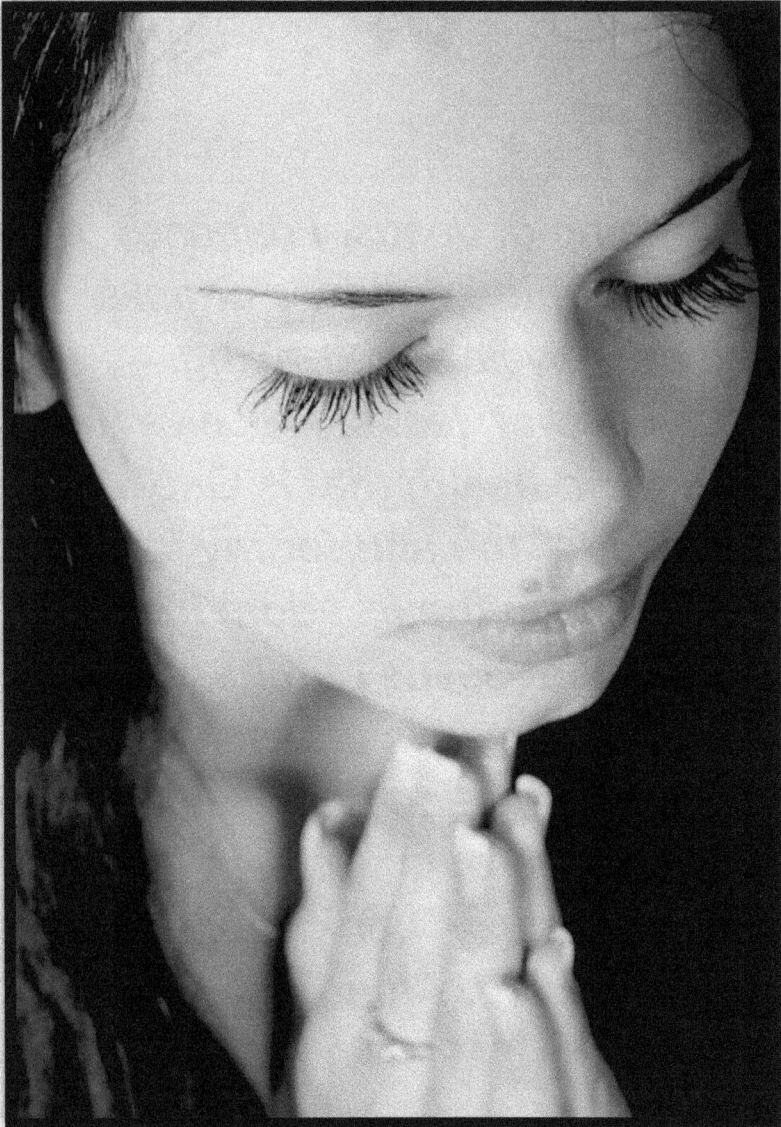

$\mathcal{T}$hank you for buying this book
and please do check out
our other
Scriptural Confessions of faith in different
topics.
Thank you again and be blessed!

http://bit.ly/2Ki0UId